LIVING WITH HIM IN VICTORY

MICHELLE BRAXTON

ii.

DEDICATION

This book is dedicated to countless families and loved ones who have been affected by HIV-AIDS directly or indirectly. It is also dedicated to those who have lost their battle with this dreadful epidemic. To those who are still in the fight, I encourage you to keep fighting. For those who are not taking wise measures to protect yourself, remember to get informed! Get tested! And Get treated! I honor the woman who gave me life, my mother, Dolores A Williams. She taught me to stand firm in my convictions and endurance in difficult times. She also taught me to accept all people, no matter their status in life. My mother had a big heart. She would take people in off the streets and care for them. She endured much to give my siblings and I a better life. She is now in the presence of the Lord. I love and miss you Mommy.

To my sister, Arzel Clark, who has taken the mantle of the hospitality gift that mommy possessed and opened your home and your table to me. You allowed me to steal away in your home during my seasons of writing this book. Thank you, "Lady" for always making me feel that I was at home. I love you to life.

To my eldest sister, Shelley Williams, aka, my second mother, who was given the caretaker's role to my younger brothers, Lawrence, Wesley, and myself. You have been a constant presence in our lives growing up even until this present time. You are the Matriarch of our family who has and still makes sacrifices to ensure that the family is well. Words cannot express my gratitude toward what you have meant to my family and I. I love you to life.

FOREWORD

After reading Michelle's book, the scripture comes to mind, "And they overcame him by the blood of the lamb and by the word of their testimony, and they did not love their lives to the death" (unwavering devotion to God unto the death). As Michelle passionately, and emphatically shares her life story, she is deliberate in declaring victory over every onslaught of the enemy, specifically the onslaught of HIV and AIDS, which was intended to end her life. Boldly declaring her testimony in written form, she fearlessly and openly declares war on the works of darkness, and wholeheartedly an unashamedly attributes her victorious living and healing to the Lamb of God: Jesus, the Christ. This book is an awesome testimonial to the power of a living Christ and promises to be a blessing and inspiration to every reader.

Reverend Dr. Joel David Rudolph
Senior Pastor
Christian Fellowship Center and
Outreach Ministries
Paterson, New Jersey

ENDORSEMENTS

It is my pleasure to have personally known Elder Michelle Braxton for over 15 years. I recognize her as a woman who has had a personal encounter with God. She is a dedicated woman of prayer and to the study of God's word, which is demonstrated by her life of integrity. Michelle's testimony is a living application of the power of God. In this book, Michelle gives you a glimpse into the reality of Luke 1:45: "And blessed is she that believed for there shall be a performance of those things which were told her from the Lord. Be unto me according to thy word…" (Luke 1:38b).

I trust that this book will inspire you to trust and believe God for great victories in your life.

Pastor Patricia Clark, Executive Pastor
Christian Fellowship Center and
Outreach Ministries
Paterson, New Jersey

Michelle is a giant in the spirit, a Prophetess of God, and a woman who has walked a walk and hence has the authority to talk the talk. Living With Him In Victory is an honest account of Michelle's life, and a victory that can be had for any believer who is anchored in Christ. Living With Him In Victory is a living testimony that negative circumstances are not the end of life but the end of one's flesh and the beginning of the Spirit of God to reign and see the supernatural power of God to deliver, heal, reclaim, and restore. Living With Him In Victory demonstrates the power behind obedience and surrender. Michelle describes event after event as she obeys, even when she did not want to. She experienced God's hand of mercy through the turmoil that bought her indescribable peace and turned her life upside down for His glory. I promise you that as you read this awe-inspiring book, it will not only rock your world, but it will challenge you, reduce you to tears, inspire you to have greater faith, and teach you some godly principles that will be great revelation and wisdom. Living With Him In Victory is indeed a book that demonstrates that in Him, there is a tremendous victory.

Christine Nelson
Founder and Project Manager
Christine Nelson Ministries
Broadcast Host Walking in Oneness
London, England

I thank God for the privilege to share my delight in support of the expanding vision of Elder Michelle Braxton. I have known Michelle from early childhood to be the woman of God that she is today. I remember sharing in her conversion about Christ and watching her grow in ministry, dynamically preaching the word of God, and praying for the needs of the people while going through great personal testing. The day of her wedding to Robert Salter gave no clue to the pain in a trial of her faith to come. However, having made a vow to her Lord, she persevered ahead, as a devoted wife, mother of two sons, and a minister in her church fellowship. I had the opportunity to pray with Robert several times before his transition, but I was not aware at the time that she had contracted "the virus". The Lord has blessed her with a special grace to give her testimony and speak words of knowledge and wisdom. Michelle comes from a long line of spiritual women that includes her great grandmother, Margaret Hayes, and grandmother, Ethel Hayes Williams, who labored in intercessory prayer for years. Several great aunts were in the ministry as well, but her grandmother, Ethel Williams, had a profound influence on her life and future. Many prophecies over Michelle's life confirmed and undergirded the fact that she is called to a great end-time work for the Kingdom of God. I believe this book will serve as a tool and weapon for the continued demise of Satan's kingdom of darkness, and to bring life, healing, and deliverance to those who read and obey. Prophetess Michelle, along with her husband, Gary Braxton, serves to confirm the scripture

Romans 1:16 "For I am not ashamed of the gospel of Christ for it is the power of God unto Salvation to everyone that believes it; to the Jew first, and also to the Greek".

Apostle Eddie Douglas Anderson
Your Father in the Gospel

Prophetess Michelle Braxton is a faithful, dedicated, consecrated, and committed anointed woman of God. I have witnessed her minister demonstratively as a servant, leader, prayer warrior, intercessor, and prolific teacher. Her very life, as she lives before men and God, is a living epistle to be read by those who witnessed her strength and courage as she forged forward during a very dark and difficult season in her life. The millions who are blessed to read this book will no doubt understand the blessedness of brokenness. In this must-read faith-filled book, Prophetess Braxton proclaims uncompromisingly the ability and willingness of God to heal, deliver and set free (from any type of bondage) those who put their trust in Him (Luke 4:18). Her riveting testimony is heartfelt, transparent, encouraging, and emboldened. Prophetess Braxton's complete confidence in the inerrant, inspired, infallible word of God is the basis on which this powerful testimony is heralded.

The Late Dr. Emma Jones
Master of Theology, Doctor of
Religious Education American
Bible College, Arkansas Faculty
member and Seminarian (25 yrs.)
Eastern Bible Institute,
Irvington, New Jersey
Director of Christian Education,
Christian Fellowship Center and
Outreach Ministries
Paterson, New Jersey

CHAPTER 1
SATAN'S PLAN

Born and raised in the inner city of Newark, New Jersey, I am the youngest girl of five siblings. Everyone was susceptible to the ills of the inner city. So, within the neighborhood, there was not a lot of backyard space.

We played in the streets, and when I was five years old, I was hit by a car. I thank God there was nothing wrong with me, and I came out unscathed. I was a victim of welfare. However, as a child, I did not realize that we were considered poor; I just knew we never could afford the popular sneakers called Pro-Keds and Converse. Being the youngest girl, my mom tried to keep things from me, and so she shielded me from a lot of things. However, parents cannot be with you all the time. I was bit by a dog and then hit by a car again; this time, I was hospitalized with a broken femur and stayed there for about a month. When I would get a visit from my paternal grandmother, whom we called Grandma Williams, she would pray with me and say, "This child is a chosen vessel." Then she would leave until the next time.

Soon after that, I was released from the hospital, dependent on crutches, and was able to do an unusual thing like put my leg behind my head. The entire neighborhood kids came over to see me do it. I became somewhat popular for a while. On occasion, they would ask me to do it, and I would. I was able to do what they could not and that made me feel a little special. I was not a girly girl, more like a tomboy. My mom would be frustrated at how quickly I could ruin my clothes. She would say "Michelle, you are so hard on your clothes." Because of this she would make sure that my clothes were durable, except on special occasions like Easter and picture day in school. Mom would put me in a dress and get my hair pressed and curled. The problem with that was that I always had a problem with perspiration so I would sweat out my hairdo. It would frustrate my mom when she would send me to the hairdresser to get my hair done, and I came home looking like nothing was done to it because my hair had drawn up. In other words, my hair was nappy.

Although I am from a family of seven, we always had someone living with us, whether it was cousins, friends, or whoever needed a place to stay. Our home was always open. My mom was compassionate toward people, so everyone was invited. Unbeknownst to her, one of them was an unsuspected molester who was a male relative. When everyone was asleep, he would visit me while I was in bed and molest me constantly at night. I dreaded going to bed at night because that is when the abuse would begin. I knew I was going to get violated by this unwanted visitor, who would take my innocence away. A child should be going to bed feeling safe and secure. I was sexually abused by someone who was supposed to protect me.

Hearing the sound that should have been my father checking in on me and making sure I was snug and given a goodnight hug, but instead, it was the other steps of terror, the footsteps of an abuser. I was only nine when the abuse started. I never told anyone at that time. Imagine sitting at the table in the morning with someone who has sexually abused you the night before, and then saying to you "good morning, can you pass the Cheerios", just having breakfast with you as if nothing happened. I never talked about it; I just buried it in my mind. I felt bad because I couldn't talk him out of doing it to me, so I lived with the secret and the shame. It did affect me as I grew up. I did not know it at the time; I was too young to process what affect it would have on me and the choices I would make later in my life. In our home, there was sometimes the physical presence of a father but not the interactive social part in our lives, because one of the issues that came with poverty was substance abuse. My father was a victim of alcoholism which kept him from engaging with the family. So, this was not the Brady bunch where there was a dad actively involved in the lives of his children. He was not there to guide us along or there for us socially or emotionally.

So, now the way I dealt with my abuse was subconsciously. I began to dress like a boy, and on occasion, I was mistaken as one. I began to wear a blue parka and jeans as my armor to protect myself from predators. I also had a terrible bedwetting problem until I was about 11 years old. There was an unusual thing that I experienced because of my abuse. I would literally bump my head until I fell asleep. Mommy used to say, "Michelle, stop it! You are going to put a hole in my wall." I couldn't stop. I tried, but I couldn't. We all deal with trauma in different ways. Now I believe that is the way I dealt with mine. I liked boys and was attracted to them, but I was afraid of them too. Because of this I did not have healthy interactions with them.

Another painful experience I had while I young was when I watched as my mother was being savagely bitten by her friend's German Shepherd. I was blamed for it and lived with the guilt and shame. I never felt good enough for most of my life. That guilt of the molestation and being blamed for my mother's attack began to foster a behavior where I tried to please people. It seemed everything I did was wrong. The feelings of guilt began shaping my life. I found myself apologizing for things for the sake of peace, even when it was not my fault. I began to walk with my head held down and could not look people in the eyes. I suffered from exceptionally low self-esteem, but people did not know because I had a quick wit. I was able to use it as a mask to compensate for my pain and insecurities.

I was quick with the tongue and could shoot you down so fast your head would spin. I was called names by the children in the neighborhood: "Chubby Checker!" "Fat Booger Nose!" All these things happened to me before I was the age of 12. I faced constant ridicule by my peers because I was a little taller for my size, but not in the least big. I began to act out in strange ways. One way was by stealing small items from the store around the corner. When I would wear my parka hood on my head, I would be mistaken for a boy; having a raspy voice did not help. The owner would always call me "boy".

Occasionally, when I went to the store with my hood on, as a way of lashing out, I would steal an item from the store. It would be an item that I did not need, such as nail polish. The devil meant for these experiences to traumatize me and shape my life for his plan. I completely understand now that these events were meant to make me a victim of my experiences and paralyze me from becoming all that God ordained for my life.

I learned that God has a plan, and so does Satan. In our childhood, Satan begins to try to impede the destiny that God has for us. He tries to use the horrible things in our past to shape us and make us conform to our experiences. Through-out those experiences, God was there, and His vessels were all around me and praying for me, although I did not know it at the time. In particular, one person who prayed was my paternal grandmother, who I previously mentioned. She would prophesy over me. I remember that as if it were yesterday.

Other people impacted my life; one was a young man that I met going to the Youth Quake Center across the street from South 8th Street School's playground. They called him brother Doug, and he worked in the office. All I knew was that there was such a glow on him, but I would refer to him as the shiny man. Even as I child, I knew something was different about him. Now I know that it was the anointing, and little did I know that he would be instrumental in my life to this very day.

Lord, I thank you for your servants who have been ordained to bring me to my purpose. May I recognize who they are and honor them for the impartations and deposits they have been called to pour into me.

During that time at the Youth Quake Center, I was taught about Jesus. Even though I was going to church, I did not clearly understand who Jesus was. I enjoyed going to the Youth Quake Center, and I learned to play pool and became good at it.

There was a Caucasian lady there named Marcy, whom I took to. She became a good friend who seemed to truly love me, which was strange to an inner-city black girl. Marcy had a love for the children in that urban area. She would take us on camping trips where I learned many Christian songs such as "Somebody Bigger Than You and I," and "Pass it On." Who knew that the time I spent there was keeping me from becoming a casualty of the streets of Newark that many of the youth my age had fallen victim to, especially with my past experiences.

I was no different from many of them; I had been molested, and I could have become promiscuous or an unwed mother. There was substance abuse all around me. I could have gotten caught up in trying to numb my pain with drugs and alcohol. But for the grace of God, there go I. I begin to love the Youth Quake Center, and it became my second home. So, because it was directly across the street from the school playground, I would eat lunch in a hurry and go there during lunch break while in school.

I wanted to know more about this Jesus, and I was introduced to Him almost every day with stories from the Bible, games, and songs.

Eventually, my mother wanted a better life for us, so she and my father bought a house in Orange, New Jersey. The time had come that we were going from the inner city to a more suburban environment at that time. Thank God we were moving from South 9th Street in Newark, New Jersey, a three-family house, to North Essex Ave. in Orange New Jersey, a one-family house with five bedrooms. The house had plenty of backyard space, a basement, and an attic. Mommy wanted to give us a better and safer life, so I could escape the streets of Newark, but I could not escape the seed of the Word that had been planted. The fruit of it was about to come forth. A hunger for God had already taken root.

The scripture says,

> "Paul planted, Apollos watered, but God gave the increase".

1 Corinthians 3:6

10

CHAPTER 2

GOD'S PURPOSE - THE VISITATION

We were excited about our new home; practically everybody had their own room which we were not accustomed to. I couldn't believe it. It was just like moving into a castle, and it was a far cry from the apartment in Newark where we were cramped. It was like something out of a fairy tale. Mommy and daddy brought a swimming pool, and it was beautiful. Relatives came over as well as our neighbors. We had cookouts almost every weekend. My mother had an excessively big heart; she always had strangers living with us to the point that they became a part of our family. I miss that house; we had exceptionally good memories there. It made up for living in Newark with those horrible experiences.

There was one experience I had that changed my life forever. In the fall, around October, I was tired and, I went to take a nap at dusk. I fell asleep and had a dream. In the dream, I was in a beautiful green field, just walking and from a distance, I heard someone call my name. "Michelle! Michelle!" I woke from the dream, ran downstairs, and asked my mother if she called me. She said, "No, Michelle,

I didn't call you!" I know that I heard a voice; it was so real to me. I can still hear that voice as if it was yesterday.

The only person I knew to call was one of God's choicest servants. She was one that I knew could explain this experience; that person was my Grandma Williams, the same woman who visited me in the hospital years ago. I was a little afraid of her. I always felt uncomfortable around her because I thought she could see through me and knew what I was doing. She was kind of scary. I called her on the phone. She had such a sweet voice and would say, "Hello dear". She called everybody "dear." I would say, "Hello, Grandma." She would always say, "I have been praying for you." Then there would be a pause on the phone, not from her but from me. Then she would say, "How may I help you?" I told her my dream. After listening to me, she recommended that I read I Samuel the 3rd Chapter in the Bible and call her back. Grandma was like EF Hutton. When she spoke, you listened. So, I did what grandma told me to do. I called her, and she confirmed what I already knew. Remember, this is the same grandma who spoke over my life in the hospital room when I got hit by a car. She said, so sweetly but firmly, "It is the Lord calling you, dear." Immediately, I felt as if my heart had fallen into my shoes. I knew it was time.

The Word of the Lord had been planted in me, and He was calling me (from the days of Marcy and the Youth Quake Center) because of Grandma's prayers and words spoken over me. She invited me to come to her church the following week for revival. Of course, I said yes. You could not say no to her. A young evangelist was scheduled to preach at the service.

The evening of the service, I was remarkably calm. During those days, devotional service consisted of singing songs and testifying about what God had done. I was accustomed to going to church, because while living in Newark, we normally did by choice. However, this time it was different; there was an excitement in the air. Now I knew it was God's presence. The guest preacher was introduced, and he looked very familiar. It was the shiny man, Evangelist Eddie Douglas Anderson, who worked in the office at the Youth Quake Center in Newark.

Evangelist Anderson was very bold and loud as he preached the Word of God. I heard the voice that was in my dream, ("You're going to get saved tonight!)."

Evangelist Anderson continued to preach, and he talked about hell and sin. I got up out of my seat and ran to the altar, even before he gave the altar call. I knelt and began to cry out to God; I was 14 years old. Then he stopped preaching and gave a formal altar call for everyone else. That night, I answered the call to salvation, and I gave my life to the Lord. I asked Jesus to come into my life and save me, and He did. I will never forget that day; it was October 16, 1976, at Calvary Baptist Church in East Orange, New Jersey. At that time, I met Jesus for the first time in my life, and I have never been the same. Romans 10:9-10 says "That if thou shall confess with thy mouth the Lord Jesus and shall believe in thy heart that God hath raised him from the dead: thou shalt be saved."

During the service, they wanted the new converts to testify of what had just happened to us. All I know is that when I began testifying, I was standing on the main floor of the sanctuary, but when I finished, I was walking out of the pulpit. I went through some terrible things in my past, but God has a purpose for my future. I would say to whoever reads this book, please don't let your past hold you hostage to your future, because everyone has a past.

However, it is up to you to decide what your future will be like. When I left the service that night, I knew that I was saved, and so did everyone else around me.

CHAPTER 3

I AM NOT ASHAMED

I did have an overly dramatic conversion. I believe it was because of what I have been called to do. Those who know me know that I am dramatic and very animated. I am also a tenacious person. Once my mind is made up about something, I am like that song: "I shall not, I shall not be moved! I shall not, I shall not be moved! Just like a tree planted by the waters, I shall not be moved!"

Yes, that is who I am. Even though who I am may have gotten on people's nerves, it helps me with my walk with the Lord. I did not have an issue, like many teens, with peer pressure. I was so glad I was saved, and I wore it like a badge. No, I did not wear a cross around my neck or carry a big family Bible to school, but I witnessed to whosoever. They called me Jesus girl, and I loved it. It gave me opportunities to preach the Word, and I did. Instead of being pressured to be like them, I challenged them to become a Christian.

For my graduation, my aunt treated me to a trip to Disney World in Orlando, Florida. My uncle drove through the south and visited all our relatives before going to

Disney World. I met my relatives and had an opportunity to witness to them. I also lead some of my cousins to the Lord. I was still a teenager, and I was witnessing to seniors and young people about Jesus. You never know when sharing the gospel if people are just tolerating what you have to say.

The Bible says in Isaiah 55:11

> "So shall my word be that goeth forth out of my mouth: it shall not return unto me void, but it shall accomplish that which I please, and it shall prosper in the thing whereto I sent it".

So, as we speak as the mouth of the Lord, we can expect things to manifest in the earth. God is always looking for a return on his Word. Yes, by that time, I had a lot of zeal. I was being taught the Word of God regularly.

My grandmother had a ministry called the Cottage Prayer Group, which consisted of a group of people hungry for the deeper things of God. They went to their churches for Sunday services and came to my grandmother for a deeper study of the scriptures and to seek the Lord. That is where I learned to pray all night. Prayer began at 7:30 pm and lasted until 6:00 am the following morning.

I experienced watching people pray, being slain in the spirit, prophesy, speak in tongues, and preach. I was the youngest one in the whole bunch. They visited different churches where Pastors welcomed them, and it started a move of God in the churches. You could call them fire starters; I was glad for such a wonderful foundation in my walk with the Lord. It has taught me how to seek the Lord in prayer and supplication.

Grandma was very instrumental in teaching me how to wait on the Lord. She would tell me to ask God questions and wait for Him to answer. She would tell me to get my Bible and a notebook and wait till God speaks to me; then, write down what He says, and date it so that when it comes to pass, I would know God spoke to me. She also said that it would help me build my faith and recognize the voice of the Lord. I can tell you that it works, and it is true.

I learned some great lessons that have helped me through some incredibly challenging times. God was faithful to bring me through every one of those storms. Prayer and intercession accompanied with the Word of God have kept me and stabilized my emotions through many painful and devastating situations. People often say: "I could have lost my mind, but God kept my mind."

Isaiah 26:3-4 says it this way

> "Thou wilt keep him in perfect peace, whose mind is stayed on thee because he trusteth in thee. Trust ye in the Lord forever for in the Lord Jehovah is everlasting strength".

The Lord hath been my strength and a strong tower. When human strength failed me, the Lord allowed me to lean on his strength to get me through. I recognized that I was eternally blessed to have quality time with a true seasoned woman of God.

Sadly, in today's society, it is hard to find older wise women in the church who are balanced in the Word and the Spirit and who are not trying to compete with the younger generation. I believe my spiritual training was vital to what was ahead of me. Only God knew what I was getting ready to endure.

We must hold fast to what we have been taught because we never know when we will need to pull from the things that we have been taught. Paul told his son in the gospel to endure hardness as a good soldier in the Lord. We are told to contend for the faith that was once delivered by the saints. We must realize that we are in a spiritual battle against the powers of darkness.

I really enjoyed going to church; I always fellowshipped with other young people, and I loved meeting new people. I was very well rounded, even though my foundation was in the Baptist church. I was Holiness and Baptist all in one. One of the places that I loved to go to fellowship was RAP. It was a gathering of saints from various denominations, and it was awesome. In the early '80s, I learned to enjoy worship songs; it was a contrast from devotional service where I would stand and worship the Lord. I have had some precious memories and wonderful experiences.

22

CHAPTER 4

GIRL MEETS MAN

As my walk with the Lord continued, I had some crushes but never serious relationships, and I had never dated.

A lot of my peers were dating and having sex. I did not even kiss a boy, although I was attracted to them. I believe that being molested caused a fear of the opposite sex, so I just pined away but never dated them. Trust me, God knew what He was doing. I believe He kept me from even more heartaches.

There was, however, one young man that I was crazy about. His name was Alphonso Davis, an exceedingly kind boy. He always treated me with respect as we walked to school together. It was, however, unrequited love; we saw each other later after High School. We talked, and I found out then that he did like me. Unfortunately, we were both afraid, and so we rejected each other. Tragically, he died several days after we met. I refused to go to his funeral; I was devastated and cried for about six months. I could not and would not eat. I was getting older and had no dating experience, but I believed that I was ready.

I was invited to attend a concert to hear a young people's choir sing. The name of the choir was Youth for Christ at New Calvary Baptist Church in Montclair, New Jersey. That night, I met a young man named Min. Robert Salter, who was the choir director. He was very animated, charismatic, and handsome. He invited me to go to IHOP with him and some of the young people. The next day, I was asked to go to Great Adventure. I went and spent my time with Robert, and there was an immediate attraction. From that day, we started seeing each other regularly. Remember, I was very inexperienced with relationships, but he was truly experienced in relationships.

I began to associate with the young people at his church very often. They were zealous, which was a complete contrast to hanging around older, seasoned women. They were my age, and we shared in common things outside the church.

I knew I was falling hard for Robert. I remember my first real kiss; I was considered a late bloomer because my first kiss was at age 19. I fell in love hard and fast; that was in August. Approximately seven months later, we were ready to get married. We were united in Holy Matrimony on February 12, 1983, a day after a major blizzard. Maybe God was trying to tell us something. If He was, we were not listening.

Have you ever wanted something so badly that you could see what was obvious? I couldn't see it. That was me. Robert was my first real relationship, and I loved him very much. He was a good husband, a provider, and dedicated to the ministry wholeheartedly. Sometimes I felt like the other woman because Robert put the church and the young people first. Because we were both still young we did not know anything about marriage; we were not equipped for what was ahead. Two years of marriage was bliss; I was a glowing bride and incredibly happy.

Isaiah 54:5-6 says

> For your Maker is your Husband the Lord of hosts is His name and the Holy One of Israel is your Redeemer; the God of the whole earth He is called. For the Lord has called you like a woman forsaken grieved in spirit, and heart sore--even a wife (wooed and won) in youth, when she is (later) refused and scorned, says your God. For a brief moment, I forsook you, but with great compassion and mercy I will gather you (to me) again'.

This scripture got my attention because I realized by that time that I had put Robert, my husband, ahead of God, and the Lord was calling me back to Him. I was extremely disappointed in my husband because I felt that he was not giving me enough attention. I felt alone, although young people always surrounded me.

Psalm 61:1-2 says

> "Hear my cry Oh God attend unto my prayer from the ends of the earth will I cry unto thee, when my heart is overwhelmed lead me to the that rock that is higher than I".

My heart was literally longing for Robert's attention; it ached with despair. Please see me, notice me, love me was my cry. When you don't fellowship with God, the one who created you for relationship, and fellowship with Him, you will seek other vices. I was like Leah mentioned in the Bible, who was always trying to get love and attention from her husband. I knew that I had put Robert ahead of my first love, which is God.

CHAPTER 5

SATISFACTION NOT GUARANTEED

I was still considered a newlywed, but a frustrated and lonely one at that point in my life. Sometimes I would stay up all night crying. So, on one occasion, during my frustration, I started to surf the channels at night. I was not looking for anything in particular but just searching because I was lonely. The first thing that caught my eye was pornography. I was shocked and embarrassed. I continued to watch, and it seemed to satisfy something, so I thought. Of course, it did not stop there. It began to relieve my frustration temporarily. I watched pornography for some time; I felt so badly, but it felt so good. By morning, of course, I was repenting, telling God I am sorry, and please forgive me! It will never happen again.

There are reports that there are more Christian women watching pornography than we realize. Can you imagine someone sitting next to you in a church that goes home and partakes in such things? Remember the height from which you have fallen! Repent and do the things you did first (Revelation 2:5).

Now, I was out of fellowship with God and had no intimacy with my husband. I was not satisfied; I was miserable; I was lonely, and now I was full of guilt. The songwriter says, "Where do I go but to the Lord?" That is what I did. I began to pray and cry out to the Lord for help! I remember those things that I was taught about God's mercy; I needed and wanted His mercy. I prayed for forgiveness. I anguished over my sin, and I asked for God's cleansing power. I asked for grace now that I had opened the door to my soul. I needed Him to close it and the power to overcome the temptation to go back. I cried unto the Lord and He heard me and delivered me from all my fears. I was forgiven, cleansed, and restored.

I thought on these scriptures:

> "Have mercy upon me, oh God, according to thy loving-kindness: according unto thy multitude of thy tender mercies blot out my transgressions. Wash me thoroughly from mine iniquity and cleanse me from my sin. For I acknowledge my transgressions and my sin is ever before me: Against thee and thee only have I sinned and done this evil in thy sight".
>
> Psalm 51:1-4a

"If we confess our sins, he is faithful and just to forgive us our sins, and to cleanse us from all unrighteousness".

1 John 1:9

I am speaking to Christians, saved folk, born again believers, and saints. We do not want people to know that we have and had struggles or issues. We like to keep that part secret because we have an image to uphold.

Meanwhile, the church continues to produce hypocrites, two-masked people, fakes, and phonies who pretend that they do not have a past or challenges post-salvation. I am not glorifying what I did, because I did it; but I am saying there is deliverance and freedom from whatever you are dealing with.

My experiences, however good or bad, taught me compassion toward people in general. Many times, as Christians, we can be so self-righteous. We forget where we came from and what we dealt with and are still dealing with, in many cases. There is forgiveness of anything you have done, no matter how dirty or guilty you feel. It is not about your feelings; it is about the truth of God's Word. Even if we feel guilty, God is greater than our feelings and knows everything (1 John 3:20). Satan will always accuse you of your sin. He is the accuser of the brethren, and it is his job to keep us preoccupied with failures.

Ephesians 2:4-5b says

> "But God, who is rich in mercy, for his great love wherewith he loved us, even when we were dead in sins, hath quickened us together with Christ".

I thank God for my experiences because they taught me brokenness and humility. I know what forgiveness is, from my sins, the nature of sin, and forgiveness from the acts or behavior of my sins. I can humbly say that I am free today. Thank God, I'm free!

The experience of watching pornography pushed me into the presence of the Lord. It caused me to develop a prayer life and return to my true love, the Lord. My passion for His presence began to intensify, and I fell in love all over again. This time, it was with the Lord. "I love the Lord because He has heard my voice and supplication" (Psalm 116:1).

CHAPTER 6

DESTINY AT THE DOOR

As I spent time with the Lord in prayer, The Spirit of the Lord began to reveal things to me. He started showing me some things about my calling. The memories of my past as a child began flooding my thoughts. What did Grandma mean when she came into my hospital room and started saying, "This child is a chosen vessel." I began to inquire of the Lord. I asked him, "Lord, is there a calling on my life, and if so, what is it?" You see, my grandma taught me years ago to ask God questions and wait for Him to answer. So, I did.

I noticed that my interest was changing. I loved to sing; my desire for prayer and the Word increased. I was one of the lead singers in the choir that my husband directed, but I was not excited about singing anymore. I wanted to spend more time in the Word. I was hungry for more of God and His presence, so I became close to a woman I met in the Cottage Prayer Group. The group consisted of men and women who were on fire for God and seeking the deeper things of God. When services were over at the churches people attended, they went to the Cottage Prayer Group's services where people sought more of God. My Grandma was the group leader, and they were invited to other churches to start revivals.

One of the young women in the group was named Sister Vickie. She was a powerful prayer warrior, and I clung to her. We attended street services, visited nursing homes, youth houses, and other churches. I watched how the Lord used her and how sensitive and open she was to the Spirit of the Lord. On the one hand, I admired her, but on the other hand, I was a little scared of her. I respected the God in her. I wanted what she had. She was able to dance before the Lord gracefully, literally like a skilled dancer. Then, she would prophesy with such power and authority. I would be in awe. Many times, we see public ministry but fail to realize their private pain.

Although I was attracted to her ministry, I remember specifically telling the Lord, "Whatever you do, don't give me that kind of gift." I remember one occasion when she began to prophesy about the children. "Pray for the children; the enemy is after our children." Then she would repeat it, "Pray for the children," and then began to sob deeply. Then she would stand up, wipe her eyes, and try to explain what the Spirit of the Lord was saying. Without any tangible proof, I believed it was the Lord, as did everybody else. So, with blind faith, we prayed for the children. Not more than a week went by when news of the killings of the children in Atlanta began to hit the airwaves. You see, God had already warned us that we needed to pray for the children and the one responsible for capturing them to be captured. The Lord answered our cry, and the killer was captured.

The hunger for the things of God grew, and I wanted more. I was apprehensive of the unknown, but I desired more of Him. As I continued to seek God fervently, He continued to affirm my calling for His purpose. So, now, I was struggling with interacting with people. I had been so wounded by those close to me that I enjoyed being with the Lord and myself more than with those who were closest to me. It was not their fault; it was just because I had trust issues. When you have suffered a lot of hurts and losses, you become apprehensive about letting someone in that close.

The journey becomes wearisome and tedious, and when you get tired in the journey, you begin to look up. David said in Psalms 3:3, "For thou O Lord art a shield for me, my glory and the lifter up of mine head."

Trouble has a way of forcing you into the presence of the Lord. I often felt like Hannah, who was provoked in her Spirit, because she had a desire for a child, but the Lord shut up her womb. There are things that God will allow to happen to us that will help birth destiny in us. He knows how to make it all work for our good. God is brilliant at interweaving everything in our lives together to create a beautiful garment.

Psalms 139:15 gives a picture of how our lives are like a quilt of different colors weaved together. We are His masterpiece like a beautiful painting with His signature on the canvas of our lives, for God is the only one that can turn trash into treasure.

2 Corinthians 4:7 says

> "But we have this treasure in earthen vessels that the excellency of the power may be of God and not us".

When we trust God, He makes what is the worst in our lives become of worth. We become a testimony of His greatness, and those who have not received Him can look and see His glory upon us.

Isaiah 60:1 says

"Arise and shine for the light is come and the Glory of the Lord has risen upon me".

Still young in the things of God and not understanding everything that God was doing in my life, I had a burning desire to live for Him more than ever. I was grateful for the discipline I had in the things of God. I was around seasoned, older saints and I loved being with them. We need this generation today to receive mentoring from the mature saints. Mentoring can keep us from the foolish mistakes we tend to make as youth. The mentor shows you a better way and can help you avoid pitfalls they have made. I believe their needs to be a Naomi-Ruth relationship.

A true Naomi can help the Ruths receive their inheritance. I have been blessed to have those types of relationships in my life. They have helped me to develop my walk with the Lord. I have learned so much being around those Saints. They showed me what a commitment to Christ is all about. They testified about pressing in and going through with the Lord. Their faith had been tested; they have been through the fire and the waters by the situations and circumstances they faced every day of their lives. There was such an inner joy and peace on them that radiated through them that you would never know they were going through circumstances and situations. They were truly living epistles.

CHAPTER 7

PRIVATE MADE PUBLIC

I had been married for a few years, and married life's troubles began to seep through from private to public. It began to show; the people within the congregation began to see the signs of trouble. Although I did my best to hide it, my countenance was showing signs of distress.

During that time, I spent a lot of time reading scriptures about women in distress and received great encouragement and revelation. I always considered myself a Hannah or Abigail. They were women in the Bible that had some very painful and public problems. I thank God for the Word of God that was such a comfort to me during those most difficult times. I can preach about these women with my eyes closed as I relate to their stories. God used them in the midst of their pain for a greater purpose than them. You see, if you are going to have power, you will have pain, but it will produce the power to do what you are called to do.

What I've have learned through my Pastor's teaching is that it is not about you. God's purpose for allowing things is greater than what you are going through right now.

Hannah agonized over not being able to have a son. God used her agony to birth a prophet, priest, and judge for the nation. Abigail was trying to save her foolish husband but ended up preserving the life of a young man that had a purpose to becoming king over all Israel, and eventually, she became his wife.

We all have a greater purpose than what we are going through. Many times, the pressures in our lives bring the purpose of our lives to the surface. As I looked back over my life, those things that seemed unbearable allowed me to bear fruit and develop my character. Your character is built from the pain and the pressure you have been through. Every great man or woman that I know has had pain and pressure in their lives. Many of our greatest commodities, such as gold and diamonds, are produced as a result of going through pressure. For each one, the pressure is applied in order for the worth and value to be at a higher value. The pressure can be heat, crushing, molding, shaping or whatever vehicle the Lord will choose to bring that which is needed to the surface, good or bad.

We are more valuable than gold or diamonds and have a greater purpose than even the precious of jewels. God has called and given to everyone a special gift and purpose.

1 Peter 2:5 says

> "You, also, like living stones, are being built into spiritual houses to be a holy priesthood, offering spiritual sacrifices acceptable to God through Jesus Christ".

It does not matter the vehicle as long as the result is the making of a godly character. The instrument God chooses is precisely the right one to help us get to our expected end.

I am reminded of a powerful revelation in the Word of God. When I was going through an exceedingly difficult time and felt the heat of the persecution, there was a scripture that God gave to me about the silver being in the hand of the coppersmith. If we can picture ourselves as the silver and Father-God as the coppersmith, we can be encouraged to know the heat of the furnace is under His control, and He will not allow the flame to be hotter than it should be. It will not burn us up, but we will stay in the fire long enough to remove the dross so that His reflection can be clearly seen.

CHAPTER 8

WHAT GOD HAS ALLOWED

During my study times, particularly when I was going through, I leaned on the Word of God as my source of comfort. As I previously stated about certain women of the Bible, one of them stood out when I needed to understand whether this was of the devil or God. Sometimes we have a misinterpretation of events because we seem to misunderstand.

One particular character in biblical history was Hannah. The Lord caused her experience. Many times, we do not know what God has allowed. We may never understand His reason, but we can rest assured that He has our best interest at heart. I have heard this saying many times: "We may not be able to trace His hand, but we can trust His heart." My pastor always says, "God will give the best to those who leave the choosing to Him."

As I continued in a deteriorating relationship, I resolved in my heart that it would be my lot. It had become strange, growing closer to the Lord and further away emotionally and physically from Robert. My ache was so deep and painful that I could not even speak about it. For me, it was so embarrassing. I loved Robert so much, and I could not understand why he was alienating himself from me. I thought maybe I was not pretty and smart enough.

I did not quite know why he turned cold and indifferent. However, I continued to stay, praying, and hoping it would get better. There always seemed to be intruders that would pull Robert away. I was still going to church regularly while he left me some weekends to go on crusades with another church.

I loved the church that I was serving, although it was very traditional; it was what we called COGIC or Church of God in Christ. I never felt that I could fit in, but I believed I was doing what a dutiful wife was supposed to do. I made the best of it. To most of the members, I seemed a little strange because of how the Lord used me in the gift of prophecy. Truthfully, I was strange, and I could not understand the way the Lord would use me at times. I do understand however that God did allow these things for a reason. Time would tell what all this would mean in the future.

I do believe that as believers, we have an advantage in everything that we go through; God can use it, if we allow him to. So, I say to the readers of this book, "Let go and let God" have His way. That means get out of the way!! You know the church lingo when somebody says I have been in the way for a long time. Sometimes that statement can be literal. So, we must say, like the song says, "Have thine own way Lord, thou art the potter, I am the clay." We must remember that God is the potter, and we are the clay. Remember that, when you want to interfere with the molding process. Clay cannot talk.

CHAPTER 9

CROSSING OVER

I remember the day Robert came to me and told me that we were leaving our church and that he found another place for us to worship. Remember when I said that he was going on crusades without me? Well, we were getting ready to be a part of that ministry. That ministry had a lot of adults our age. Can I be honest? I did not want to go. I struggled with the transition, and I consulted with one of the mothers of the church that I attended; she said she would pray with me.

I knew in my heart that I was going to the new church with my husband and children. So, when the mother told me the word from the Lord, this is what she said the Lord said: "This move will be more beneficial for you more than it will be for him." Wow, such a strange word I was hearing but never a word spoken so accurately though I did not understand it fully. I trusted the word from mother. So, I prepared myself to move.

We began attending services there; we did not immediately join, but we attended almost everything. I loved the atmosphere of worship and the Word, but I was still struggling with separation anxiety. One reason I struggled was because Robert already had established a relationship with the other ministry, and I had not, although I had met the pastor previously at a banquet. He was the guest preacher, and I loved his ministry the first time I heard him. I didn't know that one day he would become my pastor. At least I had already experienced his ministry and now knew who he was and what I would become a part of.

Do not be afraid of crossing over; there is a promise land awaiting you. Although the new land may seem like you are lost in the translation, you will soon discover the new language for the new land, and you will become part of a whole new tribe. Joining Christian Fellowship Center and Outreach Ministries under the leadership of Pastor Joel David Rudolph Sr., an Apostle in the Lord's Church, was one of the wisest choices I ever made.

It may not have made sense then, and most of what God tells us does not always make any sense at the time, but thanks be to God, who always causes us to triumph. I know the transformation that ministry has made in my life. If you know that God has set you in a house of worship, my warning to you is don't move from the place of your covering that will protect, provide, and perfect that which concerns you. It may cause you to abort your purpose or lose your very life and believe me, I have seen both happen to people who left the fellowship they were called to.

48

CHAPTER 10
WHO IS THIS STRANGER?

As my passion for the things of God increased, a strange thing started to happen within my marriage. There was an unwelcomed visitor that began to undermine my marriage and relationship with my husband. I began to notice he spent more time out then he did home. I felt like a stranger in my own house. My presence seemed to irritate Robert. He was not the Robert that I fell in love with and married.

I began to notice that the people who came in and out of Robert's life were leaving a deposit when they left. Robert's mood began to change toward me and the church that I followed him to. However, I remembered mother's words; she said, "This move will benefit you more than it will him." I became a stranger. Robert started spending less time with me, and if we happened to be in a public place, I felt as though I was intruding on Robert and his company. I became the unwelcome stranger, but I was his wife and the mother of his children.

How did this happen? I would ask myself. As I pondered the question, I realized a root of bitterness had sprung up in Robert, and the one he was fellowshipping with also had resentment and bitterness toward leadership. Neither of them dealt with their issues, and it began to contaminate every relationship and everything they attempted to do. That spirit began to prey on the innocent and others who had similar issues in the church. Unfortunately, Robert was a pawn and eventually became a victim.

When you have a wounded spirit that has not been healed by the oil of God's anointing, the devil waits for an opportune time to inflict and harass you, and you will be subconsciously operating out of your wounded spirit. That spirit will take such hold of you through that open door, and it will become so intertwined with your personality that you will have a hard time being able to distinguish the person from the spirit. Believe me when I tell you that spirits are real, and they need a body to work through.

Hebrews 12:15 warns us of this:

> "See to it that no one comes short of the grace of God; that no root of bitterness, springing up causes trouble, and by many be defiled".

We don't realize that a wounded spirit can fester and cause sickness in the body resulting in the development of many diseases; in some cases, this has been proven to be caused by unforgiveness.

Some patients have had to release a time in their past where they were wounded and had to forgive which helped them in their recovery and healing process from their illnesses. I am only telling you what I've seen with my own eyes.

If you have been hurt, abused physically, sexually, mentally, or psychologically by anyone, you have the power to rewrite the story. In other words, rewrite your story. Joseph, mentioned in the Bible, had to rewrite his story. He could have become bitter over his brothers' mistreatment of him, but he did not. He allowed God to deal with them, and he moved on to fulfill God's purpose, which included forgiving his brothers.

I know that forgiveness is a choice. You do not have to feel it or wait for some emotion to come over you; just forgive. Forgiveness does not mean that you agree with the one who victimized you. What it does mean is that you agree with God's Word which says, "Vengeance is mine I will repay." God will take care of you. He will give you the grace to go through the process of forgiveness; you do not have to stay stuck in a place of unforgiveness.

Let us visualize a person who is alive, and a dead body tied to them. First of all, you are carrying around a very heavy load called dead weight, and then that load starts to weigh you down, which affects your walk. Not only that, the dead body starts to stink. That stench gets into your clothes and eventually, your skin. Then it begins to infect you and defile you because a dead body breeds all sorts of bugs and maggots. They start crawling all over you, then the decomposition of the body begins to rub into your skin, and you become infected and eventually, you will reek of the stench of death in your talk and your walk. Pretty graphic, huh? Well, that is good. I want you to see a clear picture of what unforgiveness can do.

You will always be nursing dead things; it is like necromancy, having a relationship with dead things. That is how the Lord showed it to me; trust me when I tell you unforgiveness is not worth the heartache and the torment it brings.

CHAPTER 11

GETHSEMANE AND HIS CALLING

You are probably wondering what this chapter is about. Let me first explain why I choose these particular places (Gethsemane and Golgotha). This is also a part of my story, but even before I was born, a man named Jesus went through both of these places. I understand our experiences can never measure up to what Jesus went through in these places. We do share in His suffering, according to the scriptures. So, I wanted to tell you about my experiences and why I decided to share this place (Gethsemane) with you.

I found myself in a lonely place. Think about a lonely place where you are left by yourself to wrestle with the will of the Father. Everyone close to you has left you by yourself. That is where I was abandoned in shear agony and distress. The only comfort and encouragement I received and was getting was through the ministers of the Lord, the angels of the Lord.

Psalms 103:20 says

"Bless the Lord O you his angels, you mighty ones who do his word, hearkening to the voice of his word".

I have discovered over the course of my life that God will send his angels to strengthen us for the journey. We are human, just like Jesus. At times, He became weary and worn; and we do get weary sometimes, but God infuses us with supernatural strength to go on. Just remember Philippians 4:13 which says, "I have strength for all things in Christ who empowers me (I am ready for anything and equal to anything through Him who infuses inner strength into me: I am self-sufficient in Christ's sufficiency)."

Notice, it is through Christ, the anointed one, that we receive strength. You need the oil of His anointing to go through whatever you have been called to go through and suffer. This comes through your place of the Gethsemane experience where the anointing oil is flowing out of you and you are being pressed out. So, let it flow, let it flow, let it flow. At that time, I felt battered and beaten up by the opposition from without and within, as I shared with you in previous chapters. Who knew there was another place awaiting me? It would be the fight of my life.

CHAPTER 12

HEADING TO GOLGOTHA

Let me begin by saying that I believe, as a student of the Word that the Bible is the inspired Word of God. I believe that the Bible and the placement of events that are recorded in it are infallible. So, I believe that there cannot be a Golgotha before a Gethsemane. Golgotha means the place of the skull. I was looking at it this way: Gethsemane prepares you for Golgotha; it is the place for the battle of the mind. We understand spiritual warfare takes place in the mind. The scripture constantly reminds us about having our minds transformed by the Word of God.

During a time of intense prayer, I was in great travail, and as I was making supplication before the Lord and crying out to Him, I heard the Lord say to me, "Michelle, it's time to go to Golgotha's Hill." Of course, I was shaken by the Spirit of the Lord saying this to me. I had never heard him speak to me so emphatically; it shook me to my core. I need to say this: I thank God for the Holy Spirit, who has come to lead and guide us into all truths. Although it sounds strange to me, I knew I was being prepared for something major. I continued to ponder these words for days and weeks. I also felt led to read the book of Job.

It is amazing how the Lord can prepare you to face adversity. I was not fearful, but I was just waiting for it, whatever it was. It was winter of 1989, and the church was in consecration. I had a doctor's appointment before prayer because Robert told me that the doctor wanted to see me. So, we all went, everybody, including a family friend. I did not know what to expect, but Robert knew.

I went into the doctor's office by myself. He told me a blood test revealed that I was HIV positive. I had no response, so he continued to share that there was no cure and eventually, I would slowly become incapacitated. I left there unable to scream or talk to Robert because my children and a family friend were in the car.

Immediately, the battle began in the mind. I was at Golgotha's Hill. God had already prepared me for what I was about to face. So, I went to church that night. I got on my knees with this secret. As I began to pray, Satan spoke clearly into my spirit and mind: "Why fast and pray? You are going to die anyway." Ignoring and pressing through in prayer, Gethsemane was foremost on my mind. I cried out to God as if my life depended on it. Thoughts were constantly bombarding my mind. You are going to die! You are going to die!

I prayed with the rest of the church. We worshipped and wept, and by the end of prayer, we were embracing each other. I know I said it before but let me say it again: it is important to be under a godly covering. I thank God for my church family. They have supported, loved, and taken care of me. I also want to honor my pastor, Joel David Rudolph, Sr. He has truly been a father to me. He supported me during the most difficult and crucial times of my life, even while he was facing adversity.

As we began to minister to one another, a woman of God (I will never forget it for the rest of my life) embraced me and said, "Michelle, I don't know what you are going through, but I see the Lord giving you a blood transfusion." Let me say this: I had not told anyone that I was HIV positive. I left the doctor's office and went right into prayer at the church. No one knew but me, the doctor, Robert, and God. The woman of God who God used was the late Elder Evangelist Mary Hunter. She was one of my Gilgal Bible School instructors, who is now resting in the presence of the Lord. I miss her so much.

58

CHAPTER 13
LIVE GIRL, LIVE

So, after you get what they called a death sentence, what do you do? Live girl, live. I was pretty numb for a while because people were dying from AIDS or complications from the virus during that time. I tried talking to Robert about it, and he would not talk, so I was screaming silently. You would think that because he infected me, he would have been attentive and loving. It drove a bigger wedge between us.

My home began to be the loneliest place. I needed an answer. What am I going to do? I shut myself in and prayed to God as if my life depended on it. I fasted, and I prayed, and I prayed, and I fasted until I was sure God answered me. The Lord said to me: "Michelle, do not take the medicine. If you take it, you will die. Stay in my presence, and you will live." I had a word from God, and I was confident in it. I know it sounds crazy, but I guess you figured it out. I am a little crazy! I am crazy about my faith in God.

That night I had a dream that I was with my godfather, Pastor Douglas Anderson. We were picking out my casket because I was preparing to die. The funeral director asked me a strange question. He asked, "When is your due date?" I responded: "Due date for what?" He said, "Due date to die?" Oddly enough, I had a paper in my hand with the date and year. I looked down on the paper, and the year and day had come and gone. I asked my Godfather, "What do I do now?" He said (almost yelling at me), "Live girl, live!"

Trouble in the marriage continued. After attending an evening service, we were driving down the parkway. I tried talking to my husband, but he became paranoid about the saints talking about him. During a special church event when there were guest preachers in town, he got so angry with me that he threw me out of the car on the highway in the cold and dark. One of the saints happened to be going that way, saw me, picked me up, and took me to a restaurant. I was so humiliated and embarrassed that I sat there the whole time with my head down, looking at my plate.

I became afraid of Robert. Shortly after the incident, I went to court to get him physically removed from the house. I decided that I was not going to live like that. I stayed at the church that he brought me to; he was attending another church. Once again, the mother's words rang in my spirit: "This move will be more beneficial to you than him."

The scripture says in Job 33:16

> "Then he opens the ears of men and seals their instruction".

So, I prepared to live. You see, God speaks to us in visions and dreams. I believe that Pastor Douglas represented the Father-God telling me to live; it is not your time to die. So, I finished Gilgal Bible School because dying was not an option. When you get a word from the Lord, hold on to it.

I went back home to live with my parents. It was comforting to be around them while I was not with Robert. My sons alternated spending every other weekend with their father and I.

I became my mother's caretaker. She had a tracheotomy and didn't trust anyone but my father and I to clean it. I was glad my Mommy was there. Suddenly, my life was about to change in a week drastically. Mommy was going in to get her tracheotomy removed. Her health was getting better. She went into the hospital for the procedure. That gave me a break.

A person with a tracheotomy needs constant watching; at any time, the hole in their throat can get clogged, and it can keep them from breathing. It can happen anytime, and it did while I was sleeping. I had to sleep lightly.

Daddy worked from 11:00 pm to 7:00 am. I worked at that time and was going to Bible school. So, mom being away was a real break for me. The procedure took a day, but they kept her for observation because Mommy had a previous heart condition.

I remember coming home from work, and it was such a weird day. I was dropping things and nervous. My boss allowed me to go home early to prepare for Mommy's homecoming. I rode the bus to work, and I kept saying what a strange day.

When I got off the bus and walked down the street, my youngest brother, Wesley, was standing across the street yelling at me and telling me to go into the house. My oldest sister, Shelley, was there on the telephone. The worst possible feeling gripped me. Mommy had died. I could not believe what I heard. This cannot be happening. Not

Mommy! All my security was being stripped away from me. Not another loss! Needless to say, I was lost in my grief and now feeling guilt only because I did not go to see her that week while she was in the hospital. It seemed as if I was losing everything I loved.

I was told to live while it seemed death was all around me; first, my marriage then my momma, but I still had my boys. My sons, Joshua and Jaeson, were still incredibly young, and they were worth living for. I enjoyed Bible school; I took four classes a semester and was taking care of my boys. I still loved Robert, but it was better that we were separated. The marriage was on life support.

A lot of people wanted me to divorce him. I tried, but it did not work. When I began to file for divorce, either I had an incompetent lawyer, or God was trying to tell me something. What I mean is that when I filed the papers, the documents would be returned with my son's name on them. So, the person that I was divorcing was my oldest son, Joshua. It happened twice. I took it as a sign that it was not the way to go. I stop pursuing the divorce and just concentrated on family and ministry. I was hoping for reconciliation, but I did not know if it was going to happen.

As I accepted the call to preach, ministry doors began to open. So, I embraced the call of God and began to walk in it. My pastor recognized the ministry that God called me to. I started teaching in the school. I loved it, and I found my passion or at least one of them. The subject that I taught was prophecy (the gift and the office). That is the area God called me to. I found joy in helping others discover their gifts and being a mentor to so many others.

Focusing on other people is good medicine. I read in a book about motivational gifts that joy comes from the acronym Jesus First, Others Second, Yourself Last. Stop concentrating on your own problems and help others through their adversity, and God will surely turn yours around. Remember, Job's captivity turned when he prayed for his friends. I mentioned my Golgotha experience earlier. I read the book of Job.

Job 42:10 says

> "And the LORD turned the captivity of Job when he prayed for his friends: also, the LORD gave Job twice as much as he had before".

I preached my initial sermon on March 20, 1995. I was determined to live my life. Although we were separated at the time, Robert came to hear my initial sermon. I did not have an outfit to preach in, so a dear sister in the Lord purchased an outfit for me. Preachers are not perfect. However, God is the only one who can take imperfection to perfect the saints.

We looked like the perfect family, but we were very dysfunctional. I remember my godfather, Pastor Douglas Anderson, gave Robert a word that night and encouraged him regarding reconciliation. If he accepted, the Lord would extend his life, but the choice was his. He would give him seven years, or seven months, or seven days.

It was an awesome night. The woman of God who mentored me years ago came to my service. She had encountered many problems in her personal life, which drove her out of the church and away from God for seven years. God restored her that night. I was honored to be used to assist in God's plan to bring restoration to a woman of God who had been so instrumental in my spiritual development.

66

CHAPTER 14
GOODBYE MY BELOVED

By this time, my life was in transition. I had a sense of contentment, but the problems in my marriage still hurt me. It is amazing how God can use you to restore others, while parts of your own life are still broken.

I continued to live separate from Robert. One weekend he called me and invited me to stay with him and the boys. It was the first time that had happened for quite some time. I went and was under the same roof for 72 hours. It was strange, I had mixed emotions. I knew that Robert and I had already grown apart. We did have a love for each other, but it seemed like I was with a stranger. We made it work for the boys' sake; so, we became a family again. However, this time, I felt like a roommate.

I noticed Robert's health had started to decline; he was having trouble with coordination. A physical therapist was coming to the house to treat him. After a while, they realized that he was not getting any better. So, they stopped treatment, which really affected Robert emotionally. I continued to be supportive and became his caretaker.

We eventually had to move because the stairs became too difficult for him to climb. So, we moved into a first-floor apartment. That was when Robert became a broken man. I saw a controlling, domineering man become a scared, broken man. For me, it was hard to see him like that, unable to do for himself. Robert began to communicate with me. Oh, how I wished for time to go back to the times when I wanted to talk, and our marriage was in trouble. I had to put aside my feelings and help and support him. I had mixed emotions of hurt, anger, betrayal, and rejection. Although I wanted to help him, I was hurting.

Most of our married life (into about the third year), I never felt wanted by Robert; now, the tables had turned. He wanted my undivided attention. Each day I had to come to myself and remind myself, "Girl, it's not about you right now."

One day Robert was lying in bed, and he called me into the bedroom. I had no idea what was next. He began to say, "I always loved you, and it was never your fault. I am sorry for what I did to you. It was never your fault; please forgive me. I always loved you." I was speechless. I was so surprised at what I heard. Do you know how many times I prayed that this would happen but not under these circumstances? Now I had to process all this. Of course, I let him know that I forgave him and still loved him, too. It was bittersweet as I watched his body betray him, and he was becoming frustrated, and there was nothing I could do but be there for him.

On a Saturday, I returned from teaching a class at our church's Bible school and was preparing to go out that evening. My youngest son noticed that Robert was not responding the way he usually did. His breathing had become shallow that day, and he was noticeably quiet. I said to my youngest son, "Let me know when he wakes up." My son said, "What if he does not wake up?" I immediately went to check on Robert. When I entered the room, he was incoherent, his breathing was shallow, and he was shaking. It was amazing how things changed seemingly so drastically. I checked his pulse, and it was very faint, and he seemed to be in a semi-comatose state. I called the ambulance, and they took him to the hospital; I accompanied him.

I always wondered how one determined that a case is grave; I knew that it was serious when they turned on the sirens. They put a mask over his face to ensure that he was getting enough oxygen; he was still breathing. It was grave, but I did not know it at the time. I waited for them to tell me something when we arrived. All they said was that they would let me know when he gets a room. There seemed to be no rooms available. They acted as if they were waiting for something to happen.

The next day, there were still no rooms available. I sat uncomfortably in the emergency room. I begin to talk to Robert. At that time, they said that he probably would not make it. So, I said to Robert, "I know we have a "Do Not Resuscitate" policy, I will not enforce it." I did not want the lingering guilt or family members saying that I let him die. So, I said to Robert, "If you want to go, you can go."

As I reflect on the first time we sat down to do our living will, Robert always was resolved not to resuscitate. He said, "When it is time for me to go, let me go!" So, I said goodbye, and he sweetly and gently passed. "Goodbye My Beloved." The love of my life was lying there so still, no heartbeat and no expression. The man I loved for 13 years was gone. The one who invited me to IHOP with the youth of his church was gone. The father of my young sons was gone. There was no more to say but "Good-Bye, My Beloved, take your rest in the arms of Jesus."

Although you might sense a person is dying, there is always the denial factor. I was numb. It felt weird like a gaping hole was left. What was I going to tell his young sons? Daddy's gone?

I became a widow and a single parent all in one day. Robert's voice had been silenced by death. Returning home from the hospital and seeing his things in the house was hard. It was an incredibly sad day. The man I lived with for over a decade was gone. Now, I have to make plans, not for a date or vacation, but a home going funeral. I have to prepare to say goodbye for now. Children can be extremely sensitive to the spirit realm more sometimes then adults. So, when my young sons saw my face, they immediately knew what had happened; their faces said it all. We wept and cried together. Robert loved and adored his sons; he was truly a doting and proud father. I am glad they have the precious memories of a daddy that adored them, and I was glad I had them.

72

CHAPTER 15

MOVING FORWARD

The Home Going service for Robert was like a Home Coming and Family Reunion all rolled into one. Young people from the church had grown up; some that were married and had children were there. The wake was the way Robert would have liked it (a concert with soloists and singing). Robert was an excellent choir director, and he loved gospel music; he was very influential in the church community where he grew up. He inspired a lot of young people's lives to stay in church and with the Lord. Now, they were coming to say goodbye to their former leader and friend. Two days of his life's celebration resulted in souls being turned back to God and many relationships restored. Robert made his mistakes just like we all do, but he repented and was restored to God, and now he is resting in the Lord.

Time is a commodity, and what we do with it is important. We must live like we are dying, which means to live each moment as if it is your last. Embrace the moments that God has given to you; it is a gift. He is the giver of life and the sustainer of it. Put your trust in Him.

Psalm 25:1-2 says,

> "Unto thee, O Lord, do I lift up my soul? O my God I trust in thee: let me not be ashamed, let not mine enemies' triumph over me".

It has been 25 years since Robert's passing, and my God has been faithful. He has made me some promises, and I am still waiting for what he has in store. I have begun to move forward, doing what I believe I have been called to do. I am walking in my destiny and fulfilling the word God spoken over my life years ago by my grandmother, aka Mother Williams, "This child is a chosen vessel of the Lord."

I decided to soak myself in God's presence and stay in His face for my spiritual well-being and lead a life of the Word, worship, and prayer, which has kept me in some trying times. I continued to be faithful to God and my local church and serve as an associate minister at the Christian Fellowship Center & Outreach Ministries. I find that helping others is a wonderful medicine for what ails you. Bringing hope to others brings hope to me. Mentoring and training others in the Lord and instructing them in the ways of righteousness is what I have been called to do.

I now understand my purpose from the days of living in Newark, New Jersey, to the present. God has proven himself to be faithful. One of my favorite verses of scripture is what David said at the end of his life: "Although my house be not so with God, yet he has made with me an everlasting covenant, ordered in all things and sure: for this is all my salvation, and all my desire, although he make it not to grow" (2 Samuel 23:5). Another translation of this verse is: "I have ruled this way, and God will never break his promise to me. God's promise is complete and unchanging; he will always help me and give me what I hope for."

Staying in God's presence is the reason I am alive today. He never promised that we would not go through anything; however, He promised that He would be with us in the midst of them. As I stay in the Word, I can see God's delivering power in my life, taking me from glory to glory and from faith to faith.

God's word continues to challenge and transform my life as I yield to His will and surrender to the process. The process has sometimes been painful, but God was there with me throughout it all. I have learned compassion and mercy from my experiences, which have greatly helped me minister to others.

CHAPTER 16

THE MAN OF MY DREAMS

I believe dreams are one of the ways God communicates with man. Throughout the scriptures, we see how important dreams are to how God prepares, protects, and prevents things from happening. When we are awake, sometimes our minds get in the way of God's voice, so He uses what we call dream language to speak to us. It happened to me.

As I was going on in the things of God, I had a dream. In the dream, I was living at on South 9th Street in Newark, New Jersey, and I was coming from a house from across the street when someone yelled out, "Michelle, your husband wants you!" And I replied, "Where is he?" And they said, "He is in your house." So, in the dream, I proceeded to go back to my home. As I was approaching the house, a medium-sized built man with straight black hair came out of the house next door, and he said, "Honey, here I am!" In the dream, I liked what I saw. Then I woke up thinking it was a spiritual meaning. I tried my best to interpret it myself; I continued on with my life, while pondering the dream in my heart.

I volunteered as an office assistant at the church. One day, I was leaving the church late. A young man saw me trying to handle all my bags. As I walked to my car, he came to help me. He continued to meet me every evening and assisted me with my bags. I noticed that he came from next door. He had been attending the same church and Bible study as well. We started talking, and I asked him where he was staying. He pointed to the mission next door from the church. We began talking after church and discovered that he had been in the midst all the time. He knew who I was.

Interestingly, I had never noticed him until that day. I began to look forward to seeing him; oddly enough, he was not my usual type. He was from Baltimore, Maryland, and he was sent up here as a last attempt of rehabilitation. After he graduated from the program, he became the staff director over the men.

We started to talk more on Sundays after church, and we sometimes sat together when we were traveling to other churches in the church van. There was a single's meeting event held, and we fellowshipped. I invited him to go out because I assumed that he asked me first. Eventually, he invited me to go out, and we started going out on weekends. I felt comfortable with him; he was a perfect gentleman. He began to share the Word on our dates. For a man who had gone through what he did, he had a lot of wisdom. I could tell that he loved the Lord. Nothing is more attractive to me than a man who loves God. This man's name was and is Gary Braxton.

Let us go back to my dream. Remember when I said that I headed back to my childhood home in my dream, and a man came outside from next door and called me Honey? Well, that is Gary's description; a man that was medium built, with straight black hair, was in my house. My house represented the house of the Lord, Christian Fellowship Center, to be exact. Again, it was what I saw in the dream.

We got permission from our leader to see one another exclusively. We began to feel that we might have a future together. Gary is about seven years older than me. He had never been married. We were told to take our time to see if we were compatible. It was great dating and getting to know one another; however, it seemed like a long time waiting for us to be together, I did not need to disclose my

HIV status to him; there was no need until I knew that the relationship would result in marriage.

The day came when Gary confessed his love to me and his desire for me to become his wife. Now, I had the daunting task of telling him everything. What was he going to say? Would he still want to marry me? He was already taking on the responsibility of becoming a stepfather to my two young sons, and now this.

I remember the day that I told him everything. I said to him, "Gary, let us go for a walk; I need to tell you something." I felt that he had the right to know everything because he confessed his true intentions for me. I needed to tell the whole truth.

How do you tell someone they may be dealing with more than they bargained for? I did not want to enter a marriage with secrets, especially possible fatal ones that can come out or harm the other person involved. To those who are reading this book, please, never enter a marriage with secrets. Tell the truth before you say I do. Take a risk; you owe it to God, yourself, and the one you plan on marrying. Marriage can expose secrets that we try to hide.

Give your loved one the right to make the decision with all the information before it causes heartache and pain.

Trying to find the words to say, I said, "Honey, I need to tell you something about me. I'm only telling you this because of your intentions toward me, and you believe that I am to be your wife. I need you to know that I have been diagnosed HIV positive." I watched his face as I told him everything. He looked perplexed, so I began educating him about what I know about transmission of the virus. I told him about the myths and the facts about HIV. There was dead silence for about 30 seconds, the longest 30 seconds of my life. Then he said, "All I know is you are my wife. That's what I know! This doesn't change a thing. I love you! I do! I love you, Michelle." Needless to say, I was speechless.

The Hebrew letter for sixteen, yod-vav signifies the hand outworking of the nail that joins two people's hearts as one. That is why I chose to talk about my love story in this chapter, which signifies love. Thinking about it makes me cry happy tears. After I talked to Gary, we embraced and left the park. He invited me out to dinner one night. We drove to a beautiful restaurant called the High Lawn

Pavilion for dinner. It was about dusk up in the hills of West Orange, New Jersey, overlooking the beautiful New York City skyline at night. We ordered dinner, and as I began to eat, Gary was on the floor, and I thought that he dropped something. He pulled out a box. I could not believe what I was seeing. Was he proposing? Oh, my God!

He proposed to me at the High Lawn Pavilion in West Orange, New Jersey (overlooking New York City) with a princess cut diamond ring. Two years later, we got married on April 28, 2001. It was a beautiful spring day, and we were surrounded by family, church family and friends. I know what it means to love and be loved unconditionally. He loves me, and he showed it by accepting and taking on a woman and everything that comes with her. That is the picture of Christ and his church; he knows we have baggage, but he loves us unconditionally, despite our baggage and conditions.

CHAPTER 17

LIVING WITH HIM IN VICTORY

I chose to end this book in Chapter 17 because the number 17 represents victories. Seventeen is also one of the Hebrew letters yod-zayin, which gives a picture of the hand outworking of spiritual weaponry, which gives us victory - which is the book's theme. I John 5:4 says, "And this is the victory that overcomes the world even our faith." My Faith has been a stabilizing force in my life. It has grounded me in my walk with the Lord. The power of God has kept my mind and emotions. My heart is fixed, and my mind is made up, because I have seen and experienced God's faithfulness in my life.

I am honored every time I get the opportunity to share my story. I was the woman of the Bible with the issue. I was also the woman bent over who had no strength to raise herself up and was left crawling on the ground because life's weight caused her to be bent over.

Most people do not know this, but I used to literally walk with my head down and bent over, but Jesus' hand reached out and grabbed me, and Jesus raised me up. When my Pastor would see me like that, he would speak to me how a father speaks to his daughter and says, "Michelle, stand up, lift your head up!" Immediately, I would raise myself up.

Now I see what the devil meant for evil the Lord turned for the good.

David said in Psalm 119:71

> "It's good for me that I have been afflicted that I might learn thy statutes".

In another version, this scripture says: "When you corrected me, it did me good because it taught me to study your law".

I learned some valuable lessons in my life. I have not been innocent in everything. The scripture says there is no one good but God (Luke 18:19). In my flesh dwells no good thing.

You see, my steps were ordered by the Lord, even my mistakes. Please do not look at me as a victim. I am victorious! You see, I know something about my God. He has been where I came from and where I am going. He knows the ending from the beginning.

The scripture says in Hebrews 4:14-16 "Now that we know what we have---Jesus, this great High Priest with ready access to God----let's not let it slip through our fingers. We do not have a priest who is out of touch with our reality. He has been through weakness and testing, experienced it all---all but the sin. So, let us walk right up to him and get what he is so ready to give. Take the mercy, accept the help."   I love this translation of these verses. It shows how closely Jesus walks with us through everything we go through. He feels what we feel, He identifies with our struggles, and He has compassion on us. That is what has carried me through all these years of trials and tribulations.

Jesus was tested in the same areas as we as humans go through. Who better to seek help from if you wanted to pass a test than the teacher who created the test? If you need help preparing, or if you want to be good at a sport and perhaps go for the gold, would you seek out those who excelled in the subject or those who failed in the subject? Would you seek out those who won games and perhaps won championships or those who lost every game? Well, Jesus won every battle. The scripture says, "He has spoiled principalities and powers and made an open show of them" (Col. 2:15). He is the one that I need on my team.

Romans 8:37 says

> "Nay, in all things we are more than conquerors through Him that loved us".

It is all about knowing something about my God; I know He loves me and wants the best for me. I know His desires for me are good and not to harm me. I know that He knows the way that I take. When you know something about the one you love, it brings you to a place of total trust, and that trust gives you peace. You are intimate with them; you know their character, their nature, and their personality.

When you look at Jesus, you see and experience the fruit of the spirit, which is love, joy, peace, long-suffering, kindness, goodness, faithfulness, gentleness, and temperance. These characteristics should operate through us as they are cultivated through time spent with the Lord, in His Word, and character development through life lessons.

My sufferings brought much pain into my life; they also brought gain.

Hannah's song in 1 Samuel 2:1 says

"My heart rejoices in the Lord; my horn is exalted in the Lord; my mouth is enlarged over mine enemies. because I rejoice in thy salvation".

Throughout those difficult times, I encouraged myself in the Lord by singing, psalms, hymns, and spiritual songs and making melody in my heart to the Lord. Praise and worship will lift you above your circumstances. It is a wonderful way to see things from a heavenly view. It heightens your awareness of God's greatness. You receive strategies during those times and words of prophecy that edify, encourage, and empower you to go forth. These are spiritual weaponry, which helps us to gain the victory.

Living does not mean you just exist, but it is choosing to be present in your own life.

A wise man once said that there's a time and a season for everything - birth, death, planting, reaping, killing, healing, destroying, building, crying, laughing, weeping, dancing, for throwing stones, and gathering stones, embracing and parting, finding, losing, keeping, speaking, love, hate, war and peace. In other words, there are different seasons of our lives, which will call for a different response (Ecclesiastes 3:1-8).

None of us are exempt from trouble; trouble will always find us. The question now is, how do you handle the trouble that finds you? I choose to respond with joy. Joy gives me the strength to fight the attacks of the enemy, however it comes. Knowing the will of God, which is the Word of God, produces that kind of joy.

I now live in the Joy of the Lord. Is every day a good day? Not always, but God is good. Does everything feel good? Of course not, but it will work out for my good; and I know that no good thing will He withhold from me if I walk upright before him (Psalms 84:11b).

You may be wondering how I am living now. What does living a victorious life with God look like? What have I gained from all this?

My Gains

- A closer and more intimate relationship with the Lord
- A confidence that comes with walking with the Lord
- Joy unspeakable and full of glory
- A greater love for His Word and revelation of God and His Word
- Compassion for all people no matter what their status is in life
- An appreciation of life no matter what comes or goes

What I've Learned

- To be present - enjoy the rain, snow, or whatever comes and goes
- Love people more than I ever had because they are God's creation
- Celebrate, dance, have fun, and realize my life is a gift from God
- Say I love you more
- Forgive quicker, even my abuser and not take myself so seriously
- Say thank you
- Laugh at myself
- Be genuinely happy for people

I also learned that I still have a lot to learn, but I am open to receive what will make me better. I'm still learning humility. "I'm learning it's not about me, but about the assignment," a quote from my Pastor, Joel D. Rudolph Sr.

My life since has been very full. I have been married to Gary for 19 years. He is still a wonderful human being. I not only love him - I like him. He fills my days with laughter, especially those hard days. My sons, Joshua Darius Salter and Jaeson Daniel Salter, have been with me through a large part of my journey. I love them so much.

Both of my children love the Lord, but they face challenges like all young adults do. I appreciate all my siblings: Shelley, Arzel, Lawrence, and Wesley. I am grateful for their love and support.

It has been over 29 years since I found out about my HIV status. I feel better now than I have ever felt.

Sometimes you can wear what you are going through, and it can age you, but God can restore what the cankerworm and caterpillar have eaten. My life is a testament to the healing and delivering power of God. As you can see, God can restore your life; where you might have lost some things, He is able to give you something better. He restored my life in every part: body, soul, and spirit.

I am currently working on my third book called WAR! Today, I can say I am living! Living With Him In Victory!

ABOUT THE AUTHOR

Elder Michelle Braxton is a member of The Christian Fellowship Center in Outreach Ministries, Paterson, New Jersey, pastored by the Rev. Dr. Joel David Rudolph Sr., an Apostle in the Lord's Church. She is recognized as and functions in the office of a Prophet. She is also called to train and equip the church on how to respond to prophetic ministry in addition to training and mentoring those who have also been called to the prophetic ministry. One of her favorite scriptures is found in Isaiah 50:4 "The Lord God hath given me the tongue of the learned, that I should know how to speak a word in season to him that is weary: he wakeneth morning by morning, he wakeneth mine ear to hear as the learned."

Michelle has been featured in the International Magazine POZ. She was featured in the July 2011 Jersey Girls edition and was also included in the December 2011 issue as one of the "100 People, Things and Ideas We Love."

Elder Braxton has also acquired training as an HIV-Aids Peer Counselor at the University of Medicine and Dentistry of New Jersey (now Rutgers University). She also received a Certificate as a Peer Educator for HIV-AIDS from the Centers for Disease Control (CDC) program called WILLOW (Women Involved in Life Learning Helping Other Women).

Elder Michelle has a powerful life story that she shares to bring faith and hope to others. She shares this story in her book entitled, "Him In Victory, Living With HIV."

Michelle resides in New Jersey with her husband of 19 years, Gary L. Braxton, along with her younger son, Jaeson Daniel Salter. Her oldest son, Joshua Darius Salter, lives in

Richmond, Virginia, with his wife, LeChelle (whom Michelle affectionately refers to as her "daughter in love"), and their daughter Charleigh Jae'l.

Contact Information

E-mail: himinvictory@yahoo.com

Mbraxton62@gmail.com